Praise for

# The Joint Kitchen

"An extraordinarily helpful book about creative thinking, describing exactly what happens with me every day when I am writing."

—ALAN TRUSTMAN, Author of *Bullitt, The Thomas Crown Affair*, Recipient of the Lifetime Achievement Award from the Cannes Film Festival

"*The Joint Kitchen* by Michael Ries is a book like none other on the creative process that blends knowledge and unfocused thought leading to "outside the box" medical inventions. Dr. Ries goes beyond explaining his thought process of discovery to a description of the "silent zone," that ushers in the alchemy of the 'Eureka' moment. Invention after invention pour out of his ability to see shapes in common objects, their natural utility and his brain's own sense of itself. His opening up to his 'silent zone' is an exact description of our brain's ability to drop into the recently discovered Default Mode Network, where many believe the deepest parts of our true sense of Self exists. This critical process is centrally involved in all creative endeavors."

—MICHAEL H. MOSKOWITZ, MD, MPH, Pain Management Specialist and Author of *Medical Cannabis: A Guide for Patients, Practitioners, and Caregivers*

"Dr. Ries is an exceptional surgeon and innovator. His lessons from the silent zones of the kitchen and the outdoors provide useful guidance for innovators and for patients regarding tapping inner creativity, and applying lessons from our everyday life experience to novel utilization. This book is a must read for anyone who may hope to improve creative thinking, and to innovate and problem solve using out of the box thinking."

—SIGURD BERVEN, MD, Professor and Chief of Spine Service, Department of Orthopaedic Surgery, UC San Francisco


"A necessary read for anyone who is considering knee or hip replacement, or anyone who wishes to become an inventor in the prosthetic field, in fact, anyone who hopes to become the next Leonardo da Vinci!"

—MICHAEL E. DAVIES, Renowned Emergency Room and Trauma Physician


"*The Joint Kitchen* presents similes of everyday events which provide solutions for complex orthopaedic problems."

—SETH GREENWALD, D.Phil.(Oxon), Director, Orthopaedic Research Laboratories, Cleveland, OH

*The Joint Kitchen*

by Michael David Ries, MD

ISBN 978-1-63393-532-7

Published by

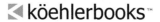 köehlerbooks™

210 60th Street
Virginia Beach, VA 23451
800-435-4811
www.koehlerbooks.com

# The Joint Kitchen

A Handbook for Orthopaedic Inventors and
Fraidy Cats Facing a Knee or Hip Replacement

Michael David Ries, MD

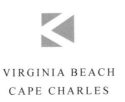

VIRGINIA BEACH
CAPE CHARLES

# TABLE OF CONTENTS

PREFACE . . . . . . . . . . . . . . . . . . . . . . . 1

I. START IN THE KITCHEN . . . . . . . . . . . . 5

    THE ORANGE . . . . . . . . . . . . . . . . 9

    THE EGG . . . . . . . . . . . . . . . . . . 18

    THE JAR . . . . . . . . . . . . . . . . . . 28

    THE CORKSCREW . . . . . . . . . . . . . 35

II. GO OUTSIDE . . . . . . . . . . . . . . . . . . 44

    THE CHAIR LIFT . . . . . . . . . . . . . 45

    THE DRY FLY . . . . . . . . . . . . . . . 56

    SNOW ON THE ROOF . . . . . . . . . . 74

    THE GARAGE . . . . . . . . . . . . . . . 81

III. FINISH THE JOURNEY . . . . . . . . . . . . 90

About the Author . . . . . . . . . . . . . . . . . . 100

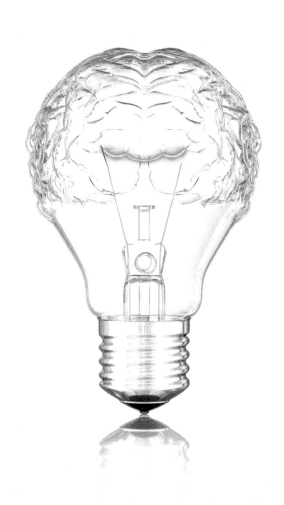

# PREFACE

THE LEFT SIDE of our brain is the logical side that figures things out. The right side of our brain is the artistic side. You probably know which one drives you. But sometimes the right and left sides of our brain talk to each other—and that's when special things happen.

Do you know the story about how Sir Isaac Newton watched an apple fall from a tree in an orchard and then he figured out gravity? He probably wasn't trying to understand why people don't fly, and he probably wasn't thinking about an apple. So it just happened.

How about Einstein? There is a story that while playing a violin he had a dream about horses racing across the sky and then thought of the theory of relativity. An entire book has been written about Einstein's dreams.

Friedrich August Kekule was a German chemist trying to figure out the structure of benzene. It seems that he discovered the ring shape of the benzene molecule after having a dream about a snake seizing its own tail.

These were very special people who did amazing things. But what makes these stories believable? They all have three elements that we are familiar with.

1.  There was awareness of a problem with no solution.
2.  An almost magical zone of silence occurred when the conscious mind was happily inactive and the unconscious side of the brain was free to think out loud.
3.  A connection occurred between conscious and unconscious thoughts that resulted in a creative idea.

So what about regular people, like you and me, and the stranger next to us? Maybe we won't save the planet, but we could have a compelling idea.

The brain is amazing. It runs without an on-off switch. Even when we are sleeping it's doing something, like making sure we breathe and our heart beats, and that we dream. If the Isaac Newton story is true, he was standing in an orchard not doing much. If the Einstein story is accurate, he was peacefully playing the violin. If the Kekule folklore is true, he had a dream, probably during sleep. So, maybe what they were doing—and when—were both important; their brain was in the right place at the right time to solve a problem.

You might wonder whether ideas come from familiar images or they just happen. When we get ideas, does it matter what we are doing? Do they come from dreams?

Will an idea surface when your head's drifting or so bored that your mind goes blank? Or, will ideas percolate if you try hard enough?

One of the above—or some combination of all three—happened to me. While doing ordinary—even mundane—repetitive activities I noticed some things about joint function that resulted in hip-and-knee-replacement inventions. In all, I have been an inventor of forty-five patents intended to improve joint-replacement technologies. In each case, they resulted from a simple question: How can we do this better?

I cannot claim that working in the kitchen, opening a bottle of wine, or slicing an orange inspired or directly influenced my inventions. But what I do know is exactly where I was and what I was doing when the ideas for these joint-replacement improvements hit me. In almost every case, I was doing something cathartic—like cooking. In each case, my mind was relaxed or I was enjoying myself. Those were my moments of inspiration. Throughout the book, I call these solution-based moments "Into the Silent Zone." It's when solutions to orthopaedic problems bubbled up or how I chose to illustrate them.

As an orthopaedic specialist, I perform hundreds of surgeries a year. So, my work is always top of mind. As with most surgeons, I always strive to improve surgical methods or technologies.

In the following pages, I write about seven surgical or technological problems I encountered, and the solution.

You will see that I use somewhat complex anatomical illustrations to show what I'm writing about, and images of basic household items or foods that either influenced my invention or help to explain it.

My intention with this book is to inspire creative thinking through common tasks, and to show in more technical detail the fruits of those brainstorms. I hope that my method for finding solutions inspires others in various professional fields. My inventions show how ordinary thoughts coming at calm moments can lead to extraordinary ideas.

I hope you enjoy my story and benefit from what I have learned.

# I

# START IN THE KITCHEN

THERE ARE A lot of great things in the kitchen. People have been eating food and preparing meals for thousands of years, and have pretty much figured out how best to do it. The best way to find out what's in the kitchen is to empty the dishwasher. This activity, which is also generally viewed favorably by spouses or housemates, requires that you identify each eating and cooking utensil in the dishwasher and place the items in cabinets and drawers containing similar things.

When you empty a dishwasher can be important. Other people in the kitchen may stake out their own personal space, usually near the refrigerator or sink or stove. So the best time to empty the dishwasher is when no one else is there, or they know what you're doing and stay out of your way. Spousal awareness of your activity may also achieve important appreciation points possibly redeemable for future personal favors.

Most of the items in the dishwasher—plates, bowls,

glasses, and silverware—are generally familiar. So, it's not too difficult to figure out where they go. After that, there may be some things that are unrecognizable, and therefore more of a challenge. These represent more advanced kitchen aids like a meat tenderizer or garlic press. You can quietly hide them in some obscure cabinet or shelf, but it's probably better to just ask someone with more knowledge and experience what it is and where it goes.

Finding a place to put the cheese grater can be difficult, because there are no other cooking items in any way similar to it. If there are no other similar utensils in any of the cabinets or drawers, you don't really have an obvious spot to put it. You could ask where it goes, but no self-respecting adult with a Y chromosome would admit such ignorance, but us Xers might. If there is no obvious spot to put something, us males might just put it anywhere.

This seemingly lackluster response is, actually, thinking outside the box. Maybe it's a small box, but still a box of conventional wisdom. Let's pretend that we put that cheese grater in some random drawer or cabinet. It's no longer in sight. Mission accomplished, correct?

Now, step back and analyze what really just happened. There is a specific reason that you put it where you did, but you probably don't know (or really care) why you chose that spot. Now you just invented something, a never-been-used-before spot to put the cheese grater. The point here is that creative thinking occurs on many levels, and we subconsciously do it every day.

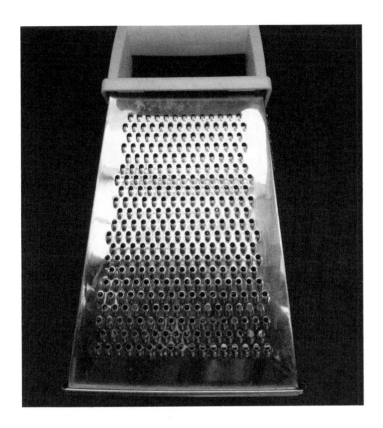

When I look at a cheese grater I see a remarkably efficient and simple tool. It is inexpensive to manufacture since holes are just punched into a flat metal sheet. Designing engineers seek to replicate the same simplicity and efficiency in surgical instruments.

Orthopaedic surgeons use a similar device to prepare bone for the acetabular socket of a total hip replacement. A "cheese grater reamer" rotates with a battery operated power tool like a drill or router to grind up and remove bone. It shapes a hemispherical cavity in the pelvis to fit the acetabular cup socket of a total hip replacement.

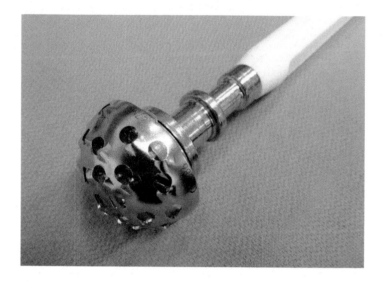

# THE ORANGE

TOTAL HIP REPLACEMENT is a wonderful treatment for arthritis. We have been doing hip replacements since the late 1960's, and the procedures and results have improved over time.

The arthritic wear of the cartilage can be seen very easily on an X-ray as narrowing of the joint surface, or space, between the hip ball and socket.

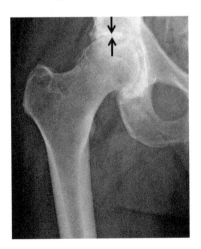

Orthopaedic surgeons are affectionately referred to as *orthopods* because of their extraordinary physical strength, genetic predisposition to understand and use carpentry tools without any prior instruction or training, and unparalleled knowledge gained through years of fixing things—like broken bones, arthritic hips, and household appliances.

A "total" hip replacement just means that you replace both the ball and the socket. There are two basic metal parts that attach directly to the bone–the stem which goes into the thigh bone (femur) and the cup or socket, which goes into the acetabulum (part of the pelvis). The artificial parts are usually made from titanium, which bone adheres to nicely. A plastic liner fits into the metal socket and a ceramic or metal ball fits onto the end of the stem so the bearing surface of the joint is formed by the ceramic or metal ball and plastic liner.

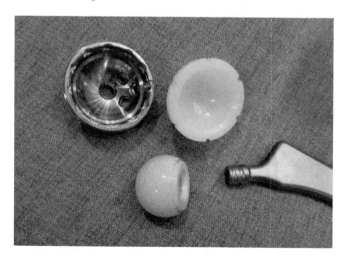

*The photo on the previous page shows a metal acetabular cup (shell), and the top right shows a plastic liner that fits into the shell. The photo below shows a pink ceramic femoral head (ball) that fits onto the femoral component (stem) at the bottom right.*

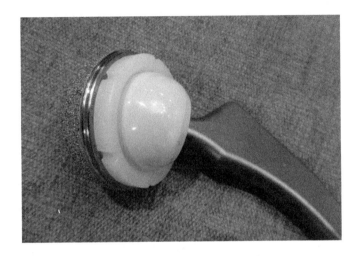

Once the parts are assembled, the replaced hip moves freely and rotates like a normal joint.

During hip-replacement surgery, the hip is dislocated (ball removed from the socket) and the acetabulum, or socket, is prepared with a "cheese grater" reamer to remove the arthritic cartilage and bone and make a smooth surface for the metal acetabular cup to fit into. The reamer creates a hemispherical cavity (half of a circle) in the bone.

Now, don't freak out at the next photo. Just imagine Julia Child and her veal chops.

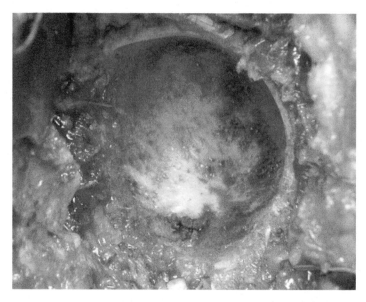

*This shows the acetabular cavity after it's reamed and the cup is ready to be put in. It might look disgusting, but not if you see it every day.*

Everyone knows that bones break when you fall on them hard enough. But bone is more like a tree limb than a rock—it bends before it breaks. In order to create a tight "press fit" of the metal cup inside the hemispherical bony cavity, the cup is slightly larger (oversized) compared to the dimensions of the reamed cavity—usually 1-2 mm. The cup is impacted into the acetabulum (with a mallet, which is a metal hammer) or "press fit," which improves stability of the cup and encourages osteointegration, or growth of bone into the outer surface of the cup, by a process that resembles fracture healing. When the reamed bony hemispherical cavity is expanded by impacting, or press fitting an oversized cup, it opens toward the rim and becomes more of an elliptical shape than a hemisphere. The cup is also hemispherical like the cavity in the bone into which it fits, but the cup is slightly larger, so it fits tightly into the bone. This means that when the cup is inserted into the bone the outer rim of the bone expands.

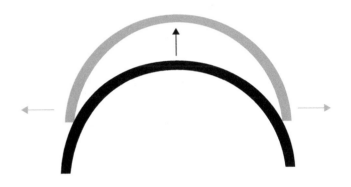

*This diagram shows how a cup (black), which is wider than the reamed acetabular cavity (blue), spreads the bone at the rim when the cup is inserted. The reamed acetabular bone is now wider at the rim than the dome. The cup is held into position when its implanted by the pressure, or tight fit, between the rim or outer part of the cup and the bone. Usually this works fine, but sometimes the cup spins out of position before the bone has a chance to bond to the cup surface, which is not good.*

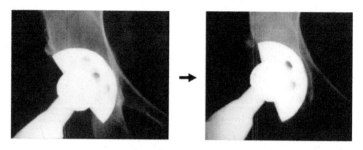

*The X-ray on the left shows the cup right after surgery, but then later on it loosened and spun out (X-ray on the right).*

## INTO THE SILENT ZONE

If you are in the kitchen you might notice that a cut orange has a similar shape to the cup and the reamer—a hemisphere.

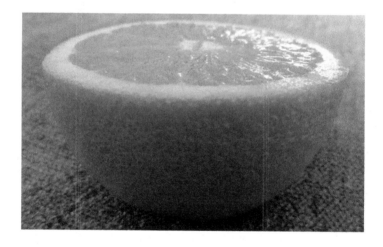

Well, the only way you can eat the orange is to cut it in half again. Then it sort of spreads apart and resembles a shape that's wider than when it started.

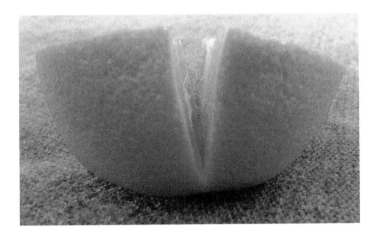

I pretty much do this every morning.

One day a friend of mine who works for a company that makes hip and knee replacements pointed out to me that two competitive companies make widened acetabular cups, which fit more tightly inside the reamed bone than hemispherical shaped cups. One of these has wider rim and is called a Dual Geometry or Dual Radius cup. Its design is protected by United States patent 4704127 and this is what the patent drawing looks like:

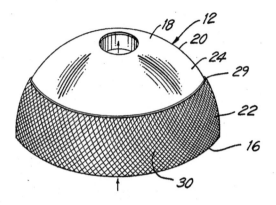

The other one has an elliptical shape. It's also patented, United States patent 5443519, and looks like this:

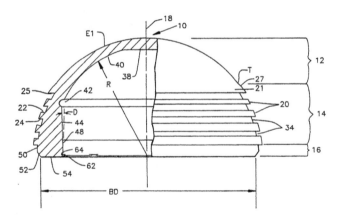

The next morning before breakfast I drew a picture of a cut orange on a napkin and sent it to my friend. Shortly after my drawing was redone professionally and became United States issued patents 5676704, 5782928, and 5879405.

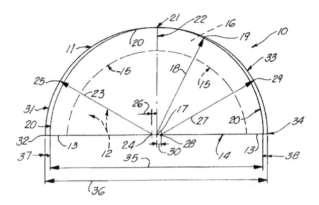

The invention worked and is named the Interfit®
*prosthesis.* (Smith and Nephew, Inc. Memphis TN)
acetabular cup.

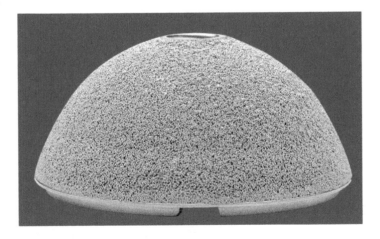

*Image reproduced with permission from Smith and Nephew,
Inc.*

# THE EGG

HIP REPLACEMENTS WORK great and many people have them now, but like anything else they can get old and wear out. If a hip replacement wears out or isn't working right, it can be fixed, which means having a redo or revision surgery. The old cup is removed and using larger reamers; a new cup is installed. The old cup was pretty much the same size as the normal or anatomic acetabulum; but the new cup is bigger. We call the revision a "jumbo" cup. It usually doesn't fit as well as the old or primary cup, so screws are used to fix it to the bone. This also works well, but there are some annoying issues with the "jumbo" cup.

## THE PROBLEM

First of all, the middle of the jumbo cup is a little higher than the middle of the smaller primary cup. This is just a geometric fact.

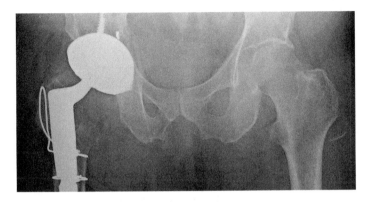

*Here is an X-ray of a jumbo cup on the left side of the picture, and a smaller normal sized hip on the right.*

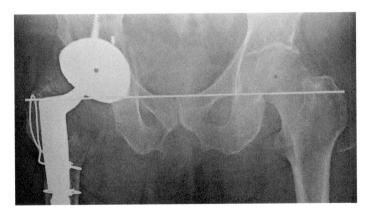

*If we put a dot in the center of each hip and a line along the bottom of the hip sockets*

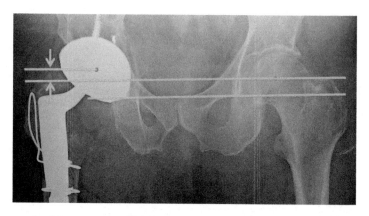

*and add some parallel lines through the center of each hip, the jumbo cup raises the center of the hip joint shown as the distance between the two arrows, which means a longer femoral prosthesis is needed to keep the legs the same length. That's not a big deal, but raising the head center also decreases the efficiency of the hip muscles so the muscles are weaker and might cause a limp. Patients who have surgery and still limp complain to their doctor, and no one likes that at all.*

The next ugly little side effect about the big cup is that it's wider than the old cup and protrudes into the front of the pelvis. If you look at the hip from the side, a cup that would be used in a primary hip replacement has bone all around it.

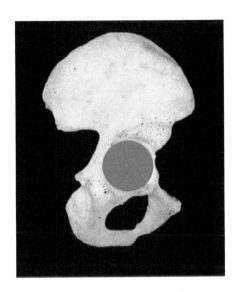

This is a side view of the pelvic bone with a blue circle showing the position and size of a normal (primary hip replacement) cup.

The jumbo cup is shown as a large green circle with a black middle part that protrudes outside of the bone toward the front of the pelvis (right side of the picture). The front of the pelvis has a lot of important body parts, one of which is the "iliopsoas" muscle.

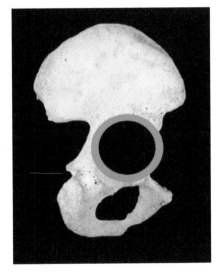

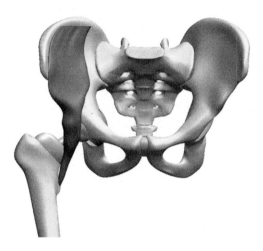

(Illustration reprinted with permission from Ries MD: The Jumbo Cup: Curtain Calls and Caveats, Seminars in Arthoplasty, 2: 155- 155, 2014 published by Elsevier)

*This is a frontal view of the pelvis with a hip replacement in it, and depicts the iliopsoas muscle in red.*

The word *iliopsoas* comes from ancient scholars who only spoke Latin. Since we don't speak Latin anymore, we now call it the *psoas* (*p* is silent so it's pronounced "soas"). The *psoas* is the main flexor muscle of the hip, so it's used when you lift up your leg to get in a car, get out of a chair, go upstairs, ski, get out of sand traps, and carry groceries into the house. After a jumbo cup is put in the hip, the *psoas* can rub on the front edge of the cup which causes tendonitis (pain) whenever the muscle is used.

There is not much we can do for *psoas* tendonitis. Physical therapy and injections sometimes help. If that doesn't work then surgery to tenotomize (cut) the tendon into two pieces stops the pain. Unfortunately this means that the muscle no longer works and the hip is weak. That's just the way it is.

## INTO THE SILENT ZONE

If you get up early in the morning, before anyone else is awake, you are on your own. The first instinct is to look in the refrigerator. Some things like yogurt and orange juice are pretty easy to consume since you don't have to cook them. Toasting a bagel is also somewhat intuitive. The next step is cooking an egg, which requires a more advanced skill set, slightly beyond operating the microwave.

To fry an egg you need to look at it in the frying pan to figure out when it's done. Sometimes it's hard to tell. You don't want to burn it, but you also want to wait long enough that the whole thing is not too gooey. The yolk is never really right in the middle.

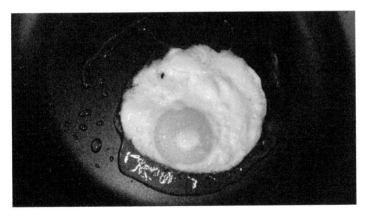

What is the egg's connection to hip replacement?

The egg resembles a jumbo acetabular cup, but the center (yolk) is at the bottom instead of the middle. If somebody made a jumbo cup with the same shape as the egg then the hip center wouldn't be elevated, which would be nice.

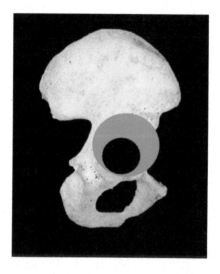

*If the new jumbo cup is put in the pelvis, the hip center looks pretty normal, but this still doesn't deal with the psoas problem.*

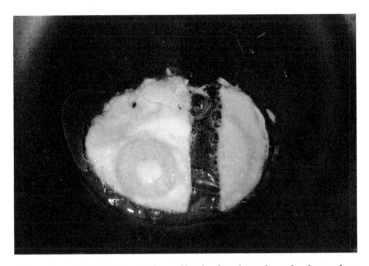

*If you have kids that eat the yolk of a fried egg last, look at what happens when they just cut off the front of the white and after you remove the cut part of the white*

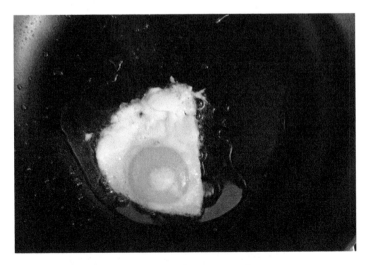

*and do the same to a new jumbo cup implant.*

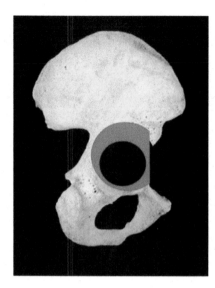

*It worked.* And so evolved United States patents 8211184 and 85704306.

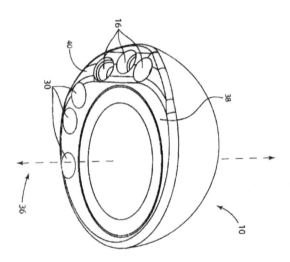

The invention is called the Restoration Anatomic Shell (Stryker Inc., Mawhaw, NJ).

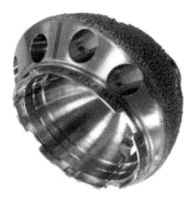

Image reprinted with permission from Stryker Corporation.
© Stryker Corporation. All rights reserved.

Now this one also happened in the morning, which is when you cook breakfast. I don't know if the fried egg directly inspired the new acetabular cup idea, but every time I fry an egg I can see its shape. It's sort of a chicken and egg story. Who knows if the egg came first or the new acetabular cup idea, but they are connected somehow.

# THE JAR

A HIP REPLACEMENT IS a ball and socket joint just like the normal hip. Once in a while, sometimes when the muscles are weak or the prosthesis is not ideally positioned, a hip replacement can dislocate (pop out of the socket), which causes incapacitating pain. Then it needs to be reduced (put back in the socket), usually under anesthesia.

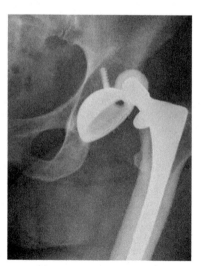

*This is an X-ray of a dislocated hip replacement.*

Occasionally this gets to be a recurrent problem and requires more surgery to fix it. One method is to use a constrained cup socket in which the ball fits into a plastic polyethylene liner. A metal ring is placed around the rim of the plastic to prevent the ball from separating. The ring makes the outer circumference of the cup smaller so it restricts hip motion, which is not great solution. Over time this mechanism often breaks.

Another way to improve the stability of the hip is to use *a dual mobility prosthesis*. Dual mobility hip replacements have a large round mobile plastic bearing that surrounds the ceramic or metal ball, and fits into a metal socket. These implants had been used for many years in Europe before they became available in the United Sates.

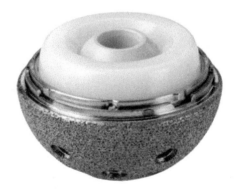

Image reprinted with permission from Stryker Corporation.

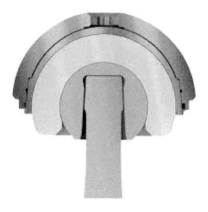

These make the femoral head (ball) bigger, which helps increase hip motion, and are difficult to dislocate, but they still can. When they dislocate, the two parts of the femoral head can separate, which is a problem. If this happens, then surgery becomes necessary to fix it. It would be nice if the dual mobility head could be constrained within the socket, preventing the two pieces from separating. If the metal liner extended past the equator, then it would constrain the head.

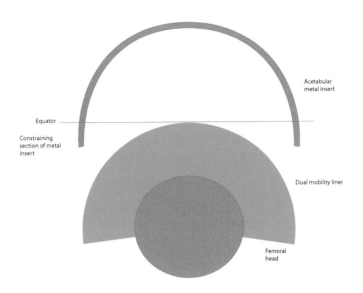

Equator

Acetabular
metal insert

Constraining
section of metal
insert

Dual mobility liner

Femoral
head

*This diagram shows how the metal insert (blue) could extend past the equator and would then hold in the dual mobility liner (green). The problem is getting the head into the liner, since the head is bigger than the cup.*

Of all the common kitchen items I routinely encounter, none influenced an invention more directly than the common canning jar. Often, they're invisible, but their simplicity is brilliant.

## INTO THE SILENT ZONE

Occasionally a jar can wind up in the dishwasher. Who knows why? Maybe one of the kids put it there because the garbage was full. Maybe your wife put it there because she wants to use it for something important. Now you've got to find the top. So now you are holding the jar top upside down to look at the inside and see if it's the right size to fit the jar. Maybe no one ever pointed this out, but the jar top has four tabs.

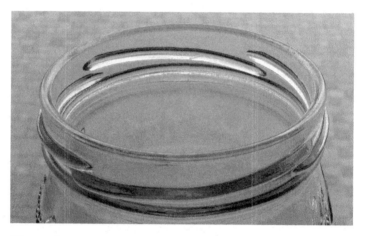

*The jar has screw threads that fit into the tabs. It's a good way to get two things to fit together.*

Unlike a nut and bolt thread, which need to be lined up with some accuracy, the jar top threads fit very easily into the jar screw threads—even if it's a little tilted.

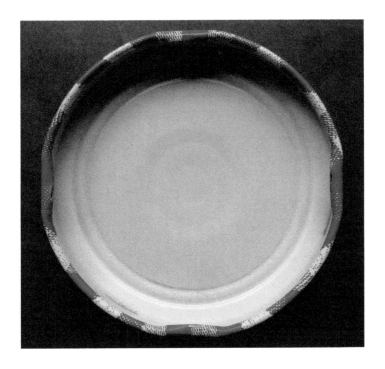

The tabs on the jar top sort of look like the rim of the constrained cup that extends beyond the equator. If the rim of the liner is more like a jar top with tabs, then the dual mobility head might be fitted with threads that could be screwed into the liner. *That might work,* I thought. The threads allow the head to be screwed in past the outer rim of the liner and then it can't separate.

So there it was right in front of my nose—a constrained dual mobility cup. This one occurred in the kitchen while holding a jar top. My patent on the devise has been filed and is pending.

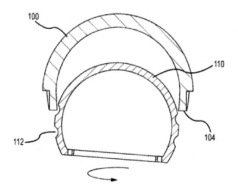

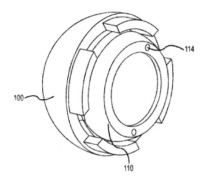

# THE CORKSCREW

KNEE REPLACEMENTS ARE a great treatment for arthritis—maybe not as good as hip replacements, but still pretty effective. There are three bones in the knee: the femur (thighbone), tibia (shinbone), and patella (kneecap). The patella is connected to the quadriceps muscle over the front of the knee. The femur and tibia are connected by ligaments, which are made of strong collagen fibers, so the knee bends like a hinge joint. It also rotates a little bit as it bends. The knee has four ligaments—two on each side (collateral ligaments) and two inside the middle of the knee (cruciate ligaments).

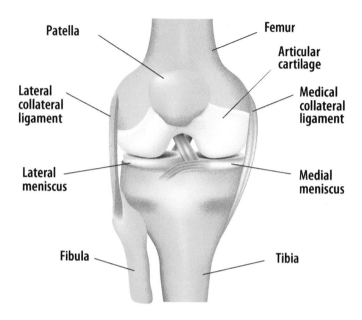

**THE HUMAN KNEE**

*When the knee is replaced, the bone surfaces are removed (cut off) and replaced with artificial (metal and plastic) surfaces.*

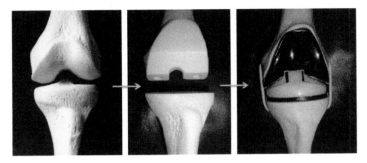

*Side view.*

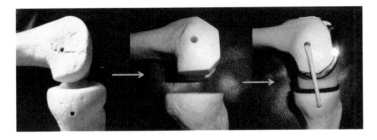

In a knee replacement, the anterior cruciate ligament is removed because it's in the middle of the knee and in the way of the replacement prosthesis. After the anterior cruciate ligament is removed the knee is less stable. A lot of people who injure their anterior cruciate ligament need to have surgery to fix it. There is also a posterior cruciate ligament. Some knee replacements retain the posterior cruciate ligament, called *cruciate retaining,* or CR.

When the two cruciates merge they twist around each other, which helps the femur rotate externally (outward) as the knee bends. This is called the *screw home* mechanism, which makes the knee fully flex and helps the quadriceps muscle to work efficiently. Unfortunately, when there is only one cruciate ligament the knee doesn't rotate normally.

The posterior cruciate ligament can be removed during knee replacement and replaced with a vertical rectangular shaped post on the tibial insert and a cam, or transverse bar, on the femoral component between the two condyles (inner and outer curved joint surfaces on the end of the femur). This is called a *posterior stabilized* or PS knee replacement.

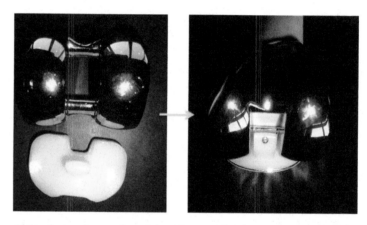

*This photo shows the white plastic tibial insert of a PS knee replacement with a rectangular shaped post sticking up. There is a horizontal metal bar between the two femoral condyles called a cam, which contacts the post and prevents posterior movement of the tibia.*

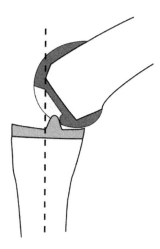

(Illustration reproduced with permission from Ries, MD. Effect of ACL Sacrifice, Retention, or Substitution on Kinematics after TKA. Orthopaedics, 30: (suppl 8);74-76, 2007 published by Slack Inc)

*This diagram is a side view through the center of a knee replacment, which shows how the cam contacts the post as the knee bends. When the cam contacts the post it stops the tibia from moving posteriorly (backwards) so this provides posterior stability to the knee and "substitutes" for PCL function.*

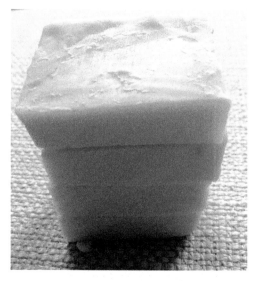

*The post is rectangular, like a stack of cut cheese squares.*

The PS knee has the cam and post for posterior stability. That's fine, but it doesn't rotate or do the screw home movement like the normal knee. If the femur doesn't rotate externally (outward) as the knee bends, then the knee may not bend fully and the quadriceps muscle loses some efficiency. It would be nice if when the replaced knee bent (flexed) it also rotated, but it doesn't. So the replaced knee works OK but not as good as the normal knee.

## INTO THE SILENT ZONE

Have you ever tried to open a wine bottle without a corkscrew? It can't be done. The corkscrew is an essential item for every kitchen and household, and deserves a prominent position in the front of the uppermost silverware drawer, so it's easy to find and easy to return to the right spot. The corkscrew rotates as it goes into the cork and unwinds as it retracts; it moves up and down and rotates.

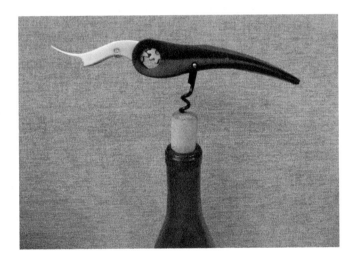

The cam of the PS knee contacts the top part of the post when the knee is relatively straight and then moves down the post as the knee bends. The post is rectangular shaped. *So how about twisting the post like a corkscrew?* I thought.

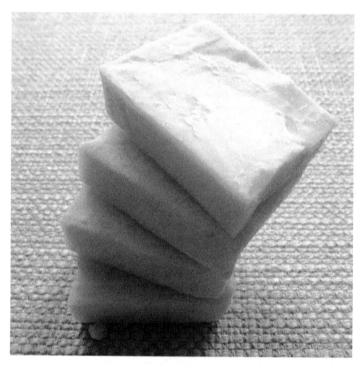

*So there it is, evolving as* US patent(s) 7356252, 7922771, 8394147, 8394148, 8398716, 8403992, 8449168, 8647389, and 9320605, *which is the Journey Total knee Replacement (Smith and Nephew, Memphis, TN).*

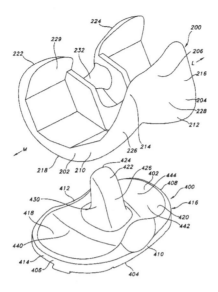

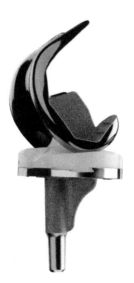

Image reproduced with permission from Smith and Nephew, Inc.

# II

# GO OUTSIDE

IN ADDITION TO the kitchen, the other "quiet spot" for reflection—at least for me—is outdoors. When there, my mind enters a tranquil state of happiness. I might get there spontaneously or when awake and doing some enjoyable activity like skiing, canoeing, biking, or fishing. Such activities require forgetting all the usual day-to-day hassles of real life.

# THE CHAIR LIFT

WHEN YOU GO outside there are usually other people doing the same thing and a lot of places where you wind up sitting next to a complete stranger. On a plane the passenger next to you may be a novice traveler compelled to convey the brutality of their flight delays and lost luggage, while an experienced frequent flyer, more likely, will avoid intrusion into your personal space in the silent hope that you will reach your destination eventually with or without personal possessions.

The nice thing about inexperienced chair lift riders is that they are blissfully oblivious to the length of the lift line, snow quality, weather, and happy to be there. A seasoned pass holder, however, might exchange valuable information about sun and snow temperature, cloud cover, and skier traffic, which is essential to find hidden terrain with unmolested soft snow. Either way, the conversation gets you up to the top.

Sometimes you wind up alone on the lift. Maybe your

ski partners exceeded the five minute rule, which is the longest anybody waits for anybody, including spouses, before getting on the lift. Sometimes you are just the only one there. When you are alone on the lift, there is not much to do, but you can see a lot. The vista of mountains, trees, rocks, and snow is only interrupted by the march of unoccupied chairlifts descending to the bottom. And your subconscious inhales both their forward progress and side to side swaying.

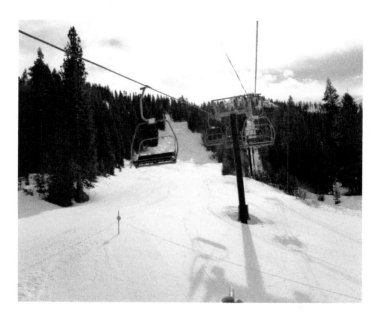

You obviously need good knees to ski down. The knee is a remarkably efficient evolutionary achievement. When the knee is straight, the femur (thigh bone) is turned inward and the tibia (shin bone) is turned outward. You can see this when you lie down in bed and your foot turns a little outward, or when watching someone run and their leg is straight.

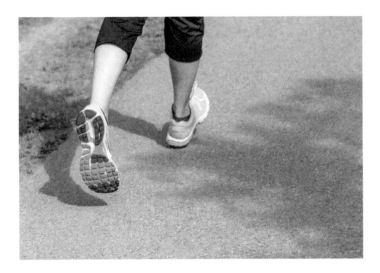

Then when the knee bends, the femur turns outward and tibia turns inward, so the foot turns in when a runner pushes off to generate more power. Some of the best sprinters are pigeon toed. When the knee bends, the femur turns outward. Another way of looking at it is that the tibia and lower leg turn inward. Did you ever wonder why your kids turn their feet in when they kneel on the floor in front of the TV? Probably not until right now. But it happens because the more you bend your knee, the more the femur rotates outward, which means the tibia rotates inward. Since your foot is connected to the tibia it also turns in.

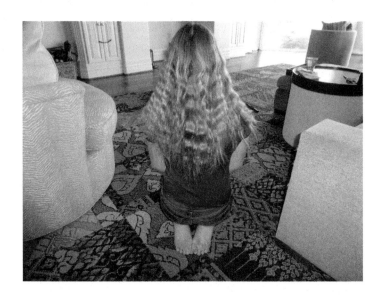

It also happens when your kids sit in front of the TV with their legs in front of them. Their hips (and femur) are turned outward, but their tibias and feet are turned inward. It looks like their feet are turned outward, but that's just because their legs are crossed.

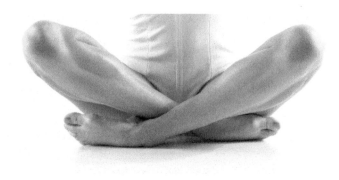

So when the young lady in the pictures grows older and walks along the *Champs-Elysees* on a crisp fall morning, the swaying of her *A*-line skirt will be driven by the same inward and outward rotations.

When you kneel with both hips rotated out and knees bent both feet still turn in which is how orthopaedic surgeons get under the sink to unclog the garbage disposal.

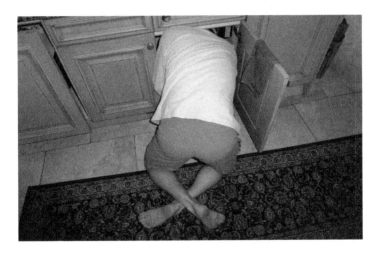

The reason the tibia turns outward when the knee is straight is because the end of the femur is tilted inward. You can't see this because your kneecap is in the front of your knee, but in knee surgery the knee is bent and the kneecap is moved to the side (temporarily) so you can see the end of the femur.

This is what it looks like. (Think of Jacques Pepin and *osso bucco*)

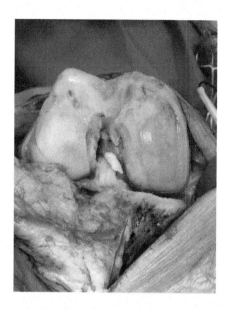

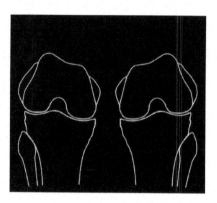

*If you draw an outline around the bone, this is what it looks like when you are sitting in a chair with both knees bent. The end of the femur is sort of tilted internally.*

## INTO THE SILENT ZONE

When looking at the empty chair lifts coming down the hill you'll see that the chair lift is shaped like the end of the femur.

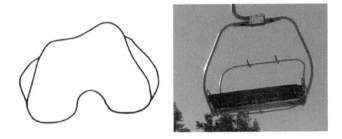

When we do a knee replacement we make a flat cut in the bone on the top of the tibia.

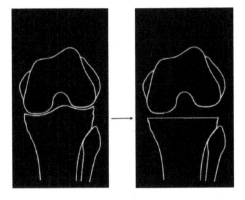

And then we need to saw off some of the bone on the front and back of the femur to fit the femoral part of the prosthesis. There are rectangular shaped cutting blocks to help guide the bone cuts.

## THE PROBLEM

The bone cuts are externally rotated to make them parallel with the cut surface of the tibia and then the prosthesis is cemented onto the cut bone surfaces, but the problem here is that the end of the femur is tilted internally so when the rectangular cutting block guide is put on the end of the femur, the externally rotated bone cuts can remove a lot of bone on the outer front part of the femur.

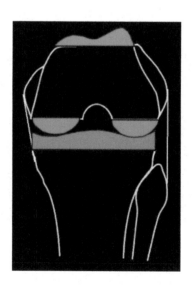

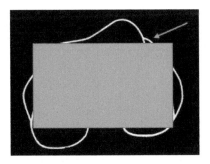

That can weaken the bone and occasionally cause a fracture, which is very bad. *So, it would be nice if we could tilt the cuts internally to fit the shape of the bone,* I thought.

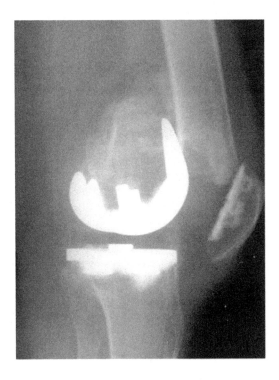

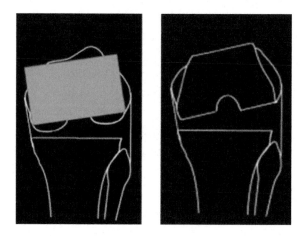

But then the gap between the two bones is trapezoidal instead of rectangular, which brought me back the chair lift.

The chairs rock back and forth. If you look at the top of one chair lift tilting inward and the bottom of the next tilting outward, and put that same shape on the end of the femur, the prostheses would still fit with the tibial component and not remove a big chunk of bone from the front of the femur.

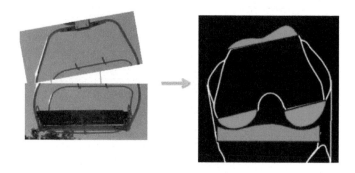

That idea resulted in US patent 5549688 and the Genesis II knee replacement (Smith and Nephew, Memphis, TN).

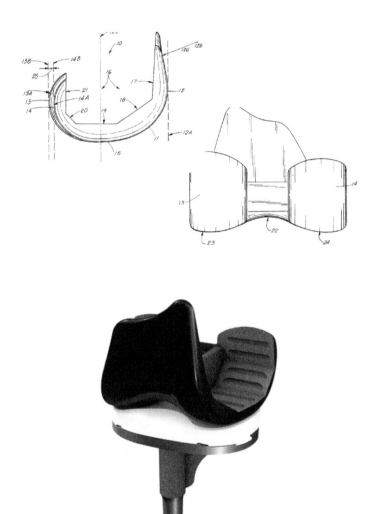

Image reproduced with permission from Smith and Nephew, Inc.

# THE DRY FLY

FLY FISHING IS about fishing. It is not about catching, but hooking them helps. When fishing, you are standing in the river, listening to the water, watching the stream, and looking at the trees and birds. It's almost meditative.

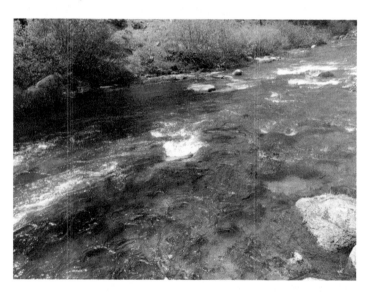

If you don't fish, shopping might be a viable alternative. Shoppers seem to explore and look at everything in the store, with or without achieving a successful purchase, and many move onto another store with little regard for time constraints. So there are peculiar similarities between fishing and shopping. There are people who like to fish and people who like to shop, but very few who like to fish and shop, except at Cabela's. And there are two fundamental differences between fly fishing and shopping; fly fishing requires instruction, while shoppers just go to the mall and start doing it instinctively. So now fly fishermen are told how to do it properly, which means there is always room to question conventional wisdom and do it *differently.*

When you are standing in the river, the current feels like a muscle pushing your thighs downstream and you have to push back. Your thigh muscle is the quadriceps, which means "having four heads" in Latin. So, there are four connected muscles that attach to the patella (knee cap).

The knee cap is a sesmoid bone which means it's small and round in the middle of the tendon at the end of the muscle. There are also some small sesmoid bones in the tendons at the base of the thumb and the big toe, but the patella is the largest sesmoid bone in the body. The patellar tendon connects the knee cap to the tibia (shin bone).

When your knee is straight, the kneecap is a little wobbly and can be moved from side to side.

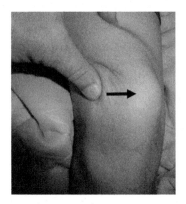 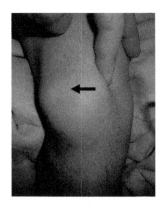

There is a reason for this. When you are standing with your legs straight, quadriceps don't do much. So, you can stand in one spot for a very long time without getting tired, like when you are waiting for a fish to inhale your fly. But as soon as you start walking and bend our knee the quadriceps muscle keeps you from falling, so you can do things like carry dirty laundry downstairs and walk back to the car to retrieve shopping items that passengers left behind. Your kneecap makes the quadriceps muscle about 20 percent more efficient. It moves down on the end of your femur as you bend your knee.

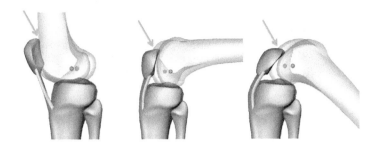

When your knee is bent, the muscle tightens up and holds the kneecap firmly in the middle. So when you bend it to get into a chair lift, or bent a lot like squatting to catch your kid's baseball, your quadriceps are stretched about as far as they can go and your knees get tired, which is why there are chairs and wheelchairs, which were invented before we had knee replacements. But when you bend your knee, remember the tibia rotates inward so it pulls the kneecap into the center of the knee.

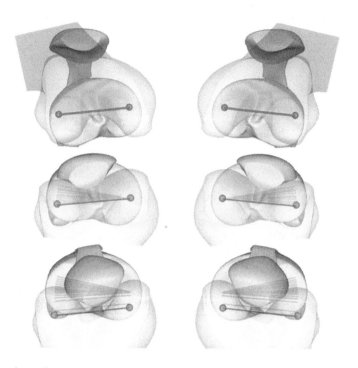

*These diagrams show what the bones do when you are standing (top of the illustration) and bend your knee into a sitting position (bottom of the illustration) if you could look down inside your knees. The red lines show how the femur rotates which pulls the kneecap sideways into the center of the knee joint*

There is a vertical groove on the front part of the femur into which the kneecap fits. If you look at an MRI, it shows the end of the femur (like the chairlift) with the kneecap in the front of the knee. The kneecap fits into a groove to keep it from slipping off the side of the knee.

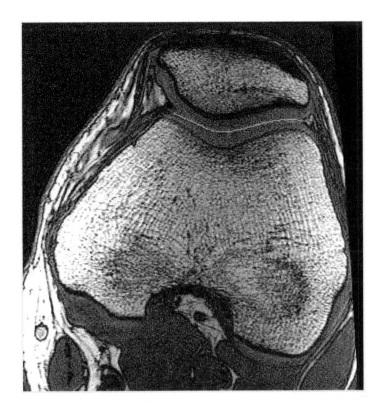

The groove can be seen as a green line on a left knee transverse MRI image where the outer part of the thigh is to the right of the image and the inner part on the left. There is also a groove in the replaced knee for the kneecap, just like a normal knee.

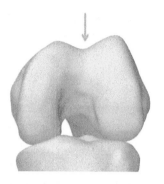
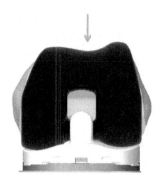

The arrow on the left shows the center of the groove where the kneecap will fit into for a normal knee. The arrow on the right shows the center of the groove for the replaced knee. When someone gets arthritis of the knee, the cartilage on the undersurface of the kneecap gets worn away and causes pain, so in a knee replacement the undersurface of the kneecap is replaced with a plastic prosthesis, which fits into the groove.

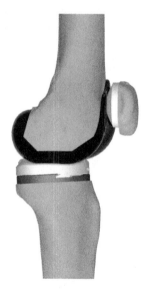

This is what it looks like from the side. There are four parts: a metal femoral prosthesis on the end of the thighbone; a flat metal tibial prosthesis on the top of the shin bone, a plastic tibial insert which attaches to the top of the tibial prosthesis; a plastic patellar prosthesis which goes on the undersurface of the kneecap.

## THE PROBLEM

The groove in the femoral prosthesis forms a track like a train track for the kneecap to slide up and down on as you bend and straighten your knee, but like anything else, the copy isn't quite as good as the original. What happens is that the kneecap tilts slightly sideways in the groove, which can be seen on an X-ray. Once in a while, it can tilt enough to be painful or even slip out of the groove.

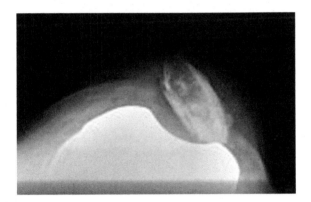

The reason it tilts abnormally is partly related to the fact that our hips are wider than our knees, more so in women, which is an aesthetic perk for the male species.

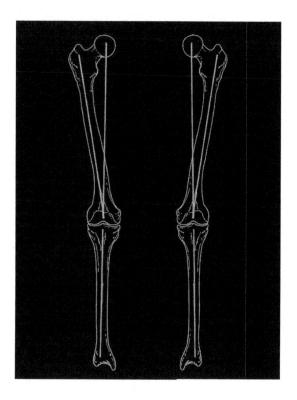

So when you are standing, the knee cap, which is part of the muscle (quadriceps), is a little more on the outside of the knee than in the middle. And remember, when you bend your knees, the shinbone (tibia) rotates inward, which pulls the kneecap toward the middle of the knee. When our knee is straight, and then starts to bend, the kneecap sort of floats down the outer side until the muscle gets tight and the shinbone (tibia) rotates inward and pulls the kneecap into the middle of the knee.

## INTO THE SILENT ZONE

There are also two general levels of fishermen—those who are perpetually learning, and fishing guides who know everything about everything and are incapable of indoor living. If you want to catch a fish you'd better understand how it lives.

Fish eat flies (insects). As far as any fisherman knows, that's why flies exist. There are two types of flies—dry flies that float on the surface of the water until they fly away, and underwater nymphs which are fetal dry flies.

Fish are like cats and only do what they have to. A high achiever cat sleeps about sixteen hours a day and takes pride in displaying his or her obesity with slow, silent movements toward a more comfortable spot. But the cat will prance into the kitchen if there is an aroma of oven roasted thinly sliced deli turkey as an alternative to bland dry commercially available conventional cat food. Fish prefer to stay in one spot and open their mouth and wait for the stream to wash nymphs (wet flies) directly into their stomach. Unless, that is, there are dry flies which hatch (evolve from wet flies to dry flies twice a day). Dry flies taste better, but require some effort for a fish to swim all the way up to the surface to eat one.

So now you want to catch a fish. There are a number of essential skills required. You need the basic equipment (fishing rod, reel, fishing line and fly on the end of the line), and fundamental skills (ability to cast the line and fly into the water upstream), advanced skills (observe the fish eating the fly, hook the fish, and reel it in), relative absence of wind blowing downstream, which prevents you from casting upstream, and an indeterminate amount of luck. The idea is to cast the fly upstream; it then starts to drift down the stream. If it drifts and "appears" like a normal healthy fly then any reasonable fish would consider it food, consume the fly, and become hooked.

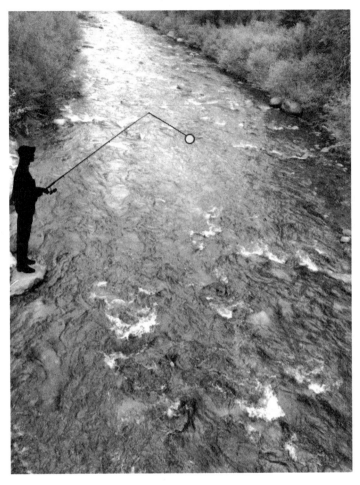

*The fly (shown as a yellow dot) and the fly line (shown as a black line) are cast upstream and then both of them start drifting downward.*

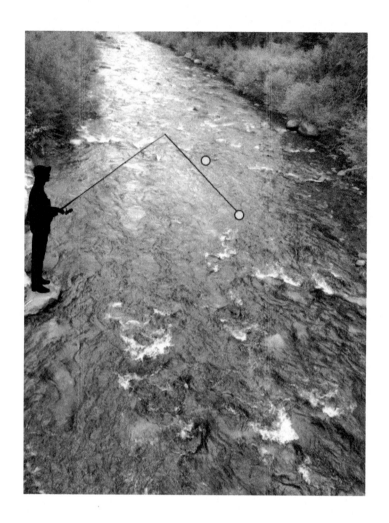

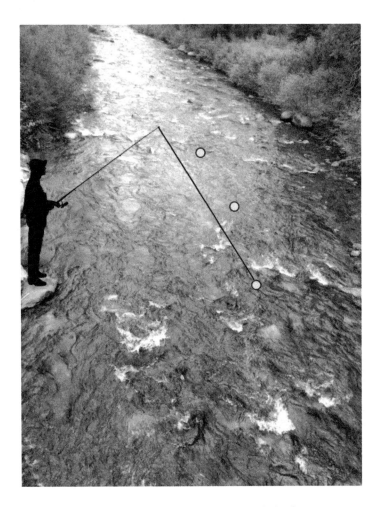

There is only so far the fly can drift before it turns sideways and heads toward shore, since it's attached to one's fishing line and is being pulled sideways across the steam. This is called the "end of the drift," and there is a zero chance of catching a fish at this point.

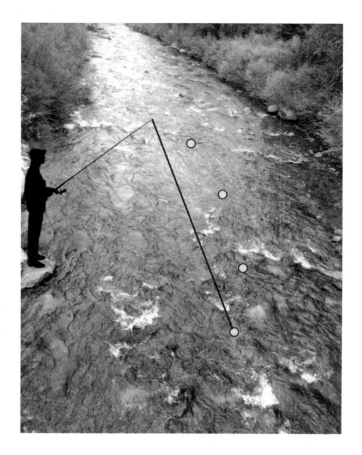

The fly line continues to pull the fly sideways across the stream toward the shore, and it's time to start all over again.

The drift is a pretty natural looking thing. The fly floats effortlessly in the stream until the end of the drift, and then the line pulls it sideways. This happens over and over, until

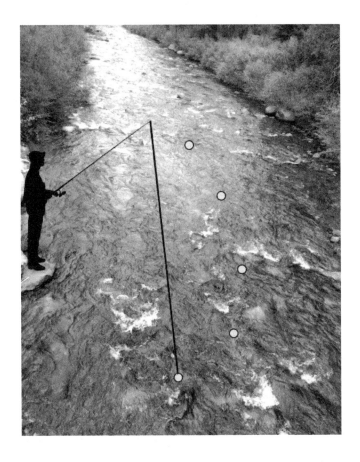

you catch your fish. So unless you are a guide, you might watch the drift many times in a hypnotic pattern. Your fly drifts straight down the current of the stream until the fly line gets tight and pulls it sideways across the stream. So, you're probably asking yourself, *What's the connection between fly fishing and drift, and bad knees?*

The path of the fly describes a *J* as it moves down the stream, similar to the path of the kneecap as it descends, guided by the groove in the femur, when the knee is bent. The tibia pulls the knee cap sideways into the middle of the knee very much like the position of the fly at the end of its drift.

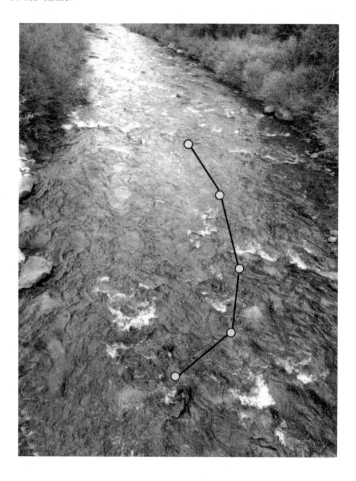

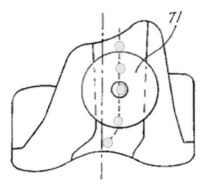

This drift pattern I described replicates the movement found in another one of my inventions—US Patent 5,825,195 and patent 5,824,105, and the Legion and Genesis II patellar groove (Smith and Nephew, Memphis, TN) This illustration came to me when I was—you got it—fly fishing.

# SNOW ON THE ROOF

YOUR KNEECAP MAY appear to be round, but it's more of an oval. Sometimes after too many years of running or skiing, and carrying suitcases up and down stairs, the kneecap cartilage can wear out, which is called *patellar arthritis*, and then it hurts when you get off a chairlift or walk down hills on the golf course. So, you might be one of those golfers in a cart and a candidate for a knee replacement.

In a knee replacement the kneecap is moved sideways and turned upside down.

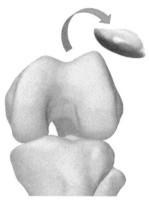

The only one who sees the upside down kneecap is an orthopod, and when the orthopod looks at the underside of kneecap every week, it always looks to him like an oval,

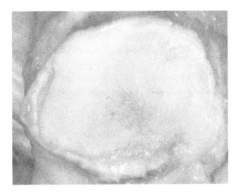

There is a ridge inside called the *median ridge* that goes down the middle.

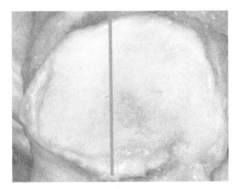

The ridge on the upside-down kneecap is pointed like the roof of a house or shed in which one stores skis and kids' sleds after dismounting the chairlift.

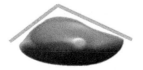 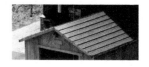

During knee replacement, a plastic prosthesis substitutes for the underside of the kneecap. So, there are three parts to the knee replacement: the femoral component, which fits on the end of the thighbone; the tibial component, which fits on the end of the shinbone; the patellar component, which fits on the underside of the kneecap.

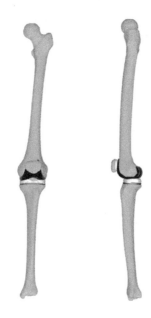

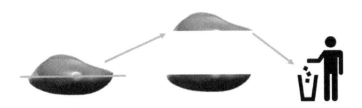

When the kneecap is replaced it is turned upside down and the top of it removed then a plastic prosthesis is cemented onto it and pegs hold it into the bone so it doesn't slide off sideways. For people with arthritis this is good, because it gets rid of all the arthritis under the kneecap.

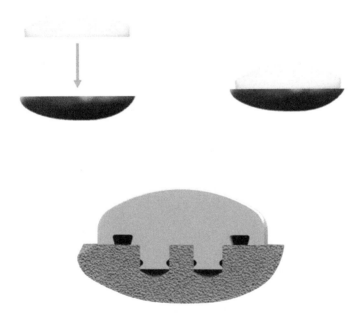

## THE PROBLEM

The kneecap is really not that big to start with, so when nearly half the bone is removed and replaced there is not much left. And a kneecap prosthesis can become worn, or the cement may loosen over time. Once in a while, it needs to be redone, which obviously is not desirable.

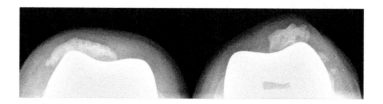

The problem with redoing the kneecap prosthesis is that half the bone is gone to begin with, and usually a little bit more, since it will have been used for a while. If you run out of kneecap bone, the quadriceps muscle no longer works. People without a quadriceps need a cane just to walk in their house.

## INTO THE SILENT ZONE

When your kids are sledding, your job is to make sure they do it in a safe place, carry the sleds up the hill, and keep them warm. When done, the kids are inside and there is usually one last walk up the hill with the sleds.

There is nothing more silent than the sound of snowflakes drifting toward the earth. The snow makes a nice clean blanket covering every house.

So, what does snowflakes and sledding have to do with kneecaps?

When I look at snow on the roof, it sort of appears like a kneecap prosthesis turned upside down, which got me thinking . . .

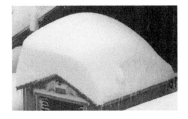 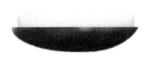

The reason we have a roof on our house is to keep the rain and snow out. There is no such thing as too much snow—there is either not enough or just enough.

So why not remove the top of the kneecap as you would snow from the roof .and then replace it with a prosthesis that looks like snow on the roof, so there is enough bone next time to redo the kneecap prosthesis?

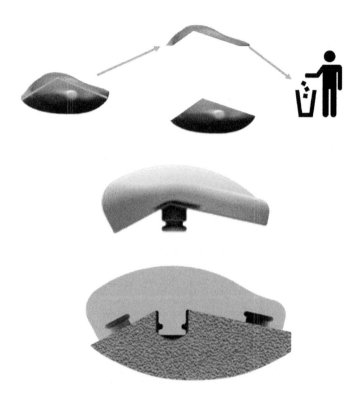

That train of thought led me to United States patent 8747478 and 8945135, and the SKYLIGN® patella.

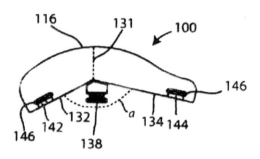

# THE GARAGE

THE NICE THING about the garage is that it's easy to find things because, ironically, no one cleans it up. Everything is just where you left it three months ago. It's also easy to find things in places that get cleaned up a lot, and to which you only go to by invitation, like the dining room or your spouse's computer desk.

It's hardest to find things in places that get cleaned up only once in a while, like the kids' rooms, where nothing is where it was last time. The garage is like the bathroom. People go there to take care of business and leave immediately after. It's a great space to experiment with ideas.

You can avoid the embarrassment of showing off your idea and finding out that it's not quite as great as you thought by going to the garage first to find out of it works. The way to do it is by making a model (prototype). You just have to find the stuff to make it. Garages often contain large items like the snow blower, golf clubs, the car, and smaller things like tools, glue, wood putty, paint cans, and ping pong balls. The garage is also an important receptacle for items which are no longer useful, but have not been useless long enough to qualify as trash that gets carried from the garage to the end of the driveway every week, like a cracked Wiffle ball or bat.

The Wiffle ball is appropriately named for a "whiff," a swing and a miss. The plastic ball is an amazing device that's hollow and has holes in the top half so it goes nowhere when you hit it with a bat, but people still can't resist the urge to try. You can cut it in half and get rid of the part with holes.

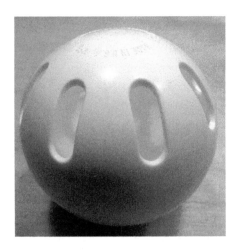

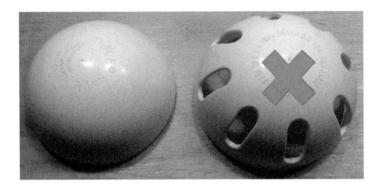

To my eye, the bottom half of the Wiffle ball is shaped like the cup socket of a hip replacement, and a ping-pong ball is about the same size as the hip ball joint, which could fit inside the Wiffle ball.

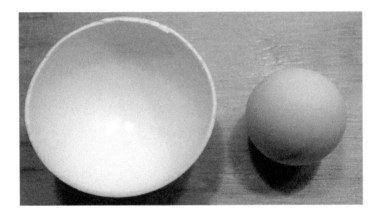

So if you look around and find some readily available wood putty, and fill the Wiffle ball with it, and then cut the ping pong ball in half (with scissors, which you can find if you look hard enough), and put it in the middle of the Wiffle ball, the whole thing looks like a hip replacement socket.

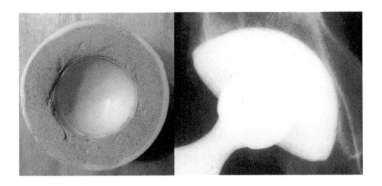

One more item is needed to complete the illustration——a hip bone to put the Wiffle ball hip replacement socket into—or something like a hip bone. This is way beyond the offerings of my garage, but fortunately you can get it on Amazon. There are plastic models of the pelvis made of an environmentally toxic non-biodegradable Styrofoam like material, which are used to try out new hip prostheses before putting them in people. And this is what they look like:

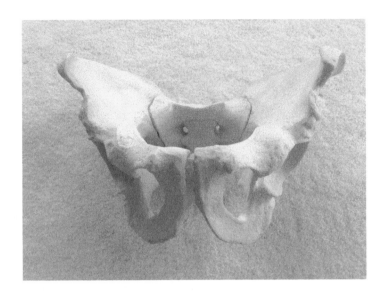

If you turn it to the side, you can see the hip socket. You may see it in your subconscious or in the Louvre as *Winged Victory*.

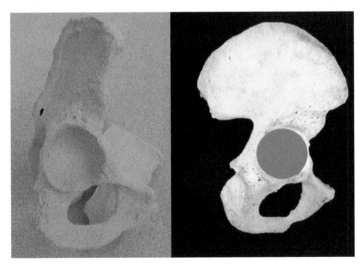

Bring your Amazon-ordered plastic pelvis to the garage and put the Wiffle ball hip replacement socket into it. It looks like a revision jumbo cup that sticks out into the front of the pelvis.

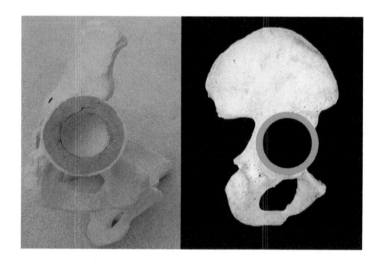

That's what we do when the old cup wears out and a new bigger cup is used to re-replace it. So, the problem we encounter here is that the oversized cup pokes into the *psoas* muscle and can cause pain when you to lift up your leg to get in a car, get off a chairlift, go upstairs, and get out of sand traps.

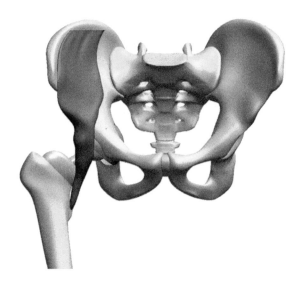

(Illustration reprinted with permission from Ries MD: The Jumbo Cup: Curtain Calls and Caveats, Seminars in Arthoplasty, 2: 155- 155, 2014 published by Elsevier)

Now remember the fried egg? The yolk is never really in the middle. So, it occurred to me, why not put the ping-pong ball at the side of the Wiffle ball instead of the middle and then cut off the egg white?

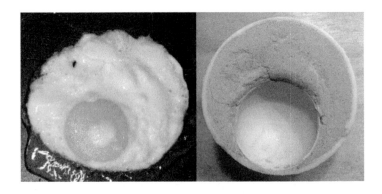

Now, do the same thing to the Wiffle ball and put it in the commercially available non-biodegradable plastic pelvis.

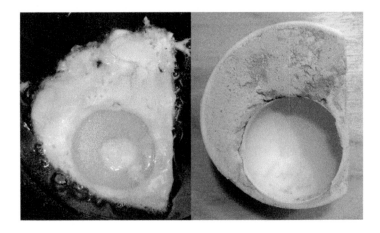

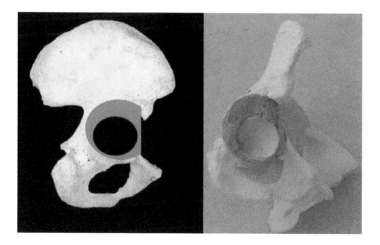

Doing so creates room for the *psoas* tendon and the hip-replacement socket is back down in its normal position. Going back to the car to retrieve shopping items that passengers left behind and carrying groceries upstairs into the house will no longer be painful.

# III

## FINISH THE JOURNEY

Transforming your idea to reality is not always easy. Who do you go to for advice about how to do it? There is also no good way to figure out if the advice is good or bad other than following it and seeing what happens. That means you have to figure out how to do it on your own which means getting out of your comfort zone. Unlike cutting an orange, frying an egg, opening a jar, uncorking a wine bottle, riding a chair lift, watching snow fall on a roof, and fishing which are familiar things that occur again and again, for me the best place to find out what to do next is to do something you never have done before. See what's still on your bucket list, like walking into an ice cave in Antarctica.

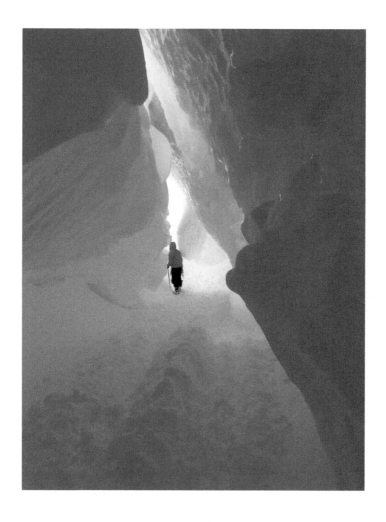

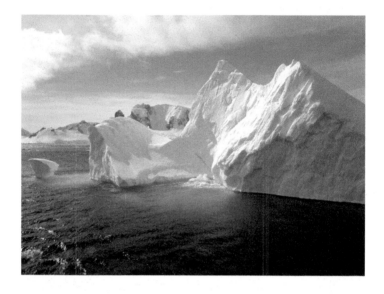

There are no roads, doors, roofs, or trees. There is just immaculate ocean, snow, and ice, which belongs to penguins.

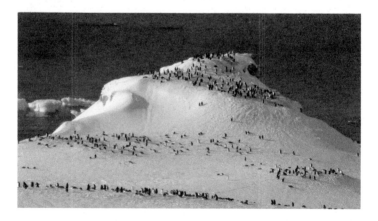

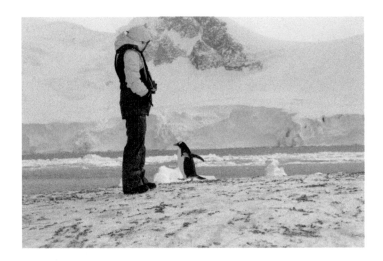

You can learn a lot from a penguin. On land they are pathetically slow and unsteady, but are the only wild creature on earth unconcerned about humans more than three times their size. The reasons penguins are at the South Pole is because polar bears are at the North Pole. So, unless polar bears figure out how to get to Antarctica (ancient Greek word for "no bear"), penguins don't need to learn how to run or fly. So, life is good from penguins.

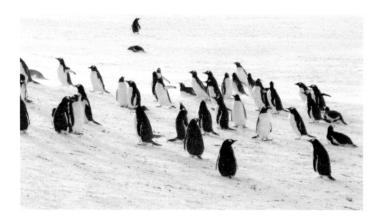

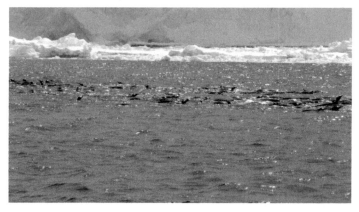

Penguins are amazingly skilled swimmers and jumpers off rocks and icebergs. This skill enables them to easily consume fish and krill (penguin term for shrimp) and escape from predatory seals in the water.

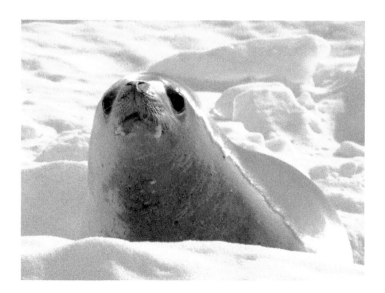

Seals look cute to us, but if you are a penguin they're ominous. So we can admire and envy the penguins, and, mostly, we can trust them. Unlike humans and the companies they work for, penguins won't steal your ideas.

Your idea (intellectual property) could be patented, which is a tangible asset, like a fish (if you are a penguin). And a penguin holding a fish in its mouth looks like both dinner and desert to a hungry seal.

Just like penguins, us humans need to protect our property from predatorial consumption, which is done by the only government agency that is self-funded and has a budget, and therefore is somewhat less dysfunctional than the rest of the federal government—the US Patent and Trademark Office.

The Patent Office offers a provisional patent, which is sort of a patent for beginners, and can be achieved by a regular person (non-lawyer), and protects the idea from theft for one year (365 days). So, now you can show your idea and see if other people think it's good.

You can show it to a big company that makes similar products. They may like it, but they may or may not need it. If your idea is "accepted"—a "yes"—then the big company, files the patent, and engages in various things that lawyers do which you never knew about before. This would generally be plan A if you don't want to spend your own money doing these things.

If your idea is rejected, a "no," and you hear "no" enough times, then it's not that your baby is ugly, but you are probably just in the right place at the wrong time. It's better to have loved and lost than never to have loved at all. No one hits a home run the first time at bat. So just go back to the kitchen and start again.

If it's neither "yes' or "no", then you are in the grey zone. If you want to upgrade your idea from the grey zone, it requires some money and some luck. You can't really rely on blind dumb luck, but it helps if you have it. The money can be yours, or come from investors. Those who invest get something in return. If other people invest a lot of money, they get a lot of your intellectual property. You and your investor friends can develop the idea some more to show it really works and then go plan A, or maybe just walk from the kitchen to the office and start up your own company.

Which way to go can depend on what your idea is about. If it's an invention for a new and improved bicycle handbrake, you need the rest of the bicycle to make it work, so it would help to partner with a company that makes bicycles. If it's an idea for an entirely new bicycle then you might need to start your own company to make them.

Money didn't come to Nero while fiddling as Rome burnt, or to Einstein while roaming in his subconscious as he played the violin. Gambling capital is another strange ramble in a country, as they say, not for old men.

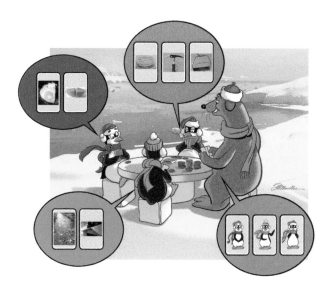

The point of all of this is that when you unleash your mind and create an item or hatch a profound idea, protect that mental brainstorm. The trademark and patent process can be cumbersome, but it is also your best friend. If you don't protect your intellectual property it is bound to be high jacked, just like a hungry seal high jacking a penguin with a fish in its mouth. But if your dream is to see your idea turn into reality it will only happen if you just do it.

# About the Author

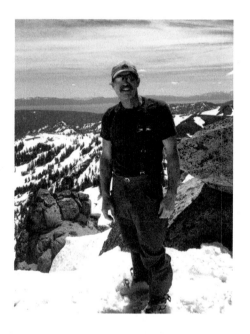

 Dr. Michael Ries is a world renowned orthopaedic surgeon. He has presented over 600 invited lectures at regional, national, and international orthopaedic educational conferences, and published over 200 peer reviewed journal articles and 50 book chapters on topics related to total hip and knee replacement. Dr. Ries is also an inventor on 45 US patents for hip and knee replacement devices.